MAKEUP
ARTIST

FACE CHARTS

FROM THE BEAUTY STUDIO COLLECTION

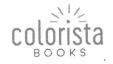

colorista
BOOKS

www.coloristabooks.com

Cover designer: Gina Reyna
Interior layout: Gina Reyna
Illustrator: Holly Christie (@avecholly)

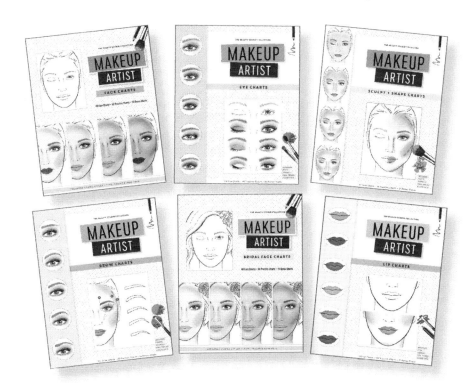

Contents

FACE CHARTS

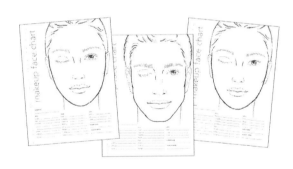

48 total face charts. Faces come with & without brows so you have the option of drawing your own.

BONUS MAKEUP CHARTS

Sample makeup charts from other books in the Beauty Studio Collection!

GETTING STARTED

This book contains practice charts, makeup charts and bonus makeup charts for hours of coloring fun! Follow the User Guide to discover tips, techniques, and how-to's to customize your makeup looks like a pro!

Color & customize your makeup charts with colored pencils, markers, crayons, even real makeup! Makeup charts include product/color logs so you can easily keep track of what you use for each look.

COLORING WITH MAKEUP

Dry makeup formulas such as powder eyeshadow, blush, bronzer & flesh-tone face powders blend easily on paper. An advantage of powder, is that it can be removed with an eraser. White erasers are recommended over colored ones as they are less likely to stain.

You may find cream & liquid products diffcult to use as they tend to apply blotchy & can leave oil stains. However, is possible to use these types of products if you apply them in thin layers. See **'Pro Tips + Tricks'**, to learn more about cream & liquid application techniques.

ABOUT PAPER TEXTURE

Paper texture or "tooth" is about how the surface of paper feels. The more tooth paper has, the rougher it will feel because it has lots of tiny bumps & grooves. Makeup face charts within this book are printed on paper with little tooth, giving it a fairly smooth texture. Now, depending on your choice of coloring material(s), you may find that some products adhere better than others.

If certain products/colors aren't applying as vibrant as you would like, consider adding some tooth to the paper. An easy ways to do this is with texture hairspray (aerosol) - simply mist the surface of the paper with a thin layer and let dry.

Another way to add tooth is with clear gesso paste.* Apply a thin even layer with a wide synthetic paint brush and let dry. Rinse brush with water immediately after use. If paper feels too gritty, gently smooth surface with fine sandpaper.

Clear Gesso by Liquitex, Artist's Acrylic or Dina Wakley is recommended.

MAKEUP APPLICATION TOOLS

When it comes to applying makeup on a chart, you'll find that smaller brushes offer more control over placement & blending. The most useful eye brushes include:

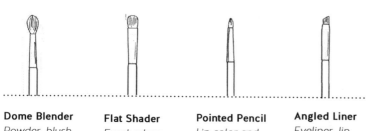

Dome Blender
Powder, blush, bronzer, contour and highlight

Flat Shader
Eyeshadow and contour

Pointed Pencil
Lip color and defining eyes

Angled Liner
Eyeliner, lip liner & defining brows

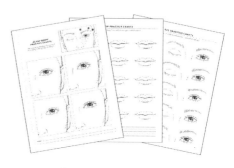

Build your skills with practice charts

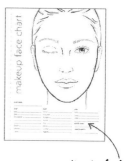

Keep track of products + colors

HOW TO BUILD A PORTFOLIO

Create your own makeup portfolio to showcase your skills & looks. All you'll need are scissors, 8.5" x 11" (3-ring) binder & clear protective sleeves. Cut along dashed line to remove makeup chart from book & put in protective sleeve.

Use binder tab dividers to categorize & organize looks by makeup styles (day, night, bridal, dramatic, smokey eyes, etc..) and/or makeup looks for various skintones (fair, light, med, tan, dark).

Alternatively, you can leave makeup charts in book and use sticky note tab labels to catergorize and organize.

Adding Skincolor

• Add any shade of skin color to a makeup chart with flesh-tone face powder and a dome blender brush.

• For smooth even results, pick up powder with brush then dab on back of hand to distribute powder evenly into the bristles. Use light circular motions to color in "skin". Repeat until you have reached your desired shade.

• Avoid whites of eyes as you shade in skin. If any makeup gets onto the eyes, use a white eraser to remove it. Alternatively, you can mask the eyeballs before you color the skin with removable tape or a thin coat of clear nail polish.

Powder Makeup

For smooth application - pick up powder with brush & dab on back of hand to distribute evenly into the bristles. Use small circular motions when blending color on paper. Repeat until you reach desired shade.

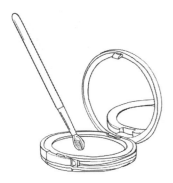

Cream + Liquid Makeup

The key to achieving the best results with cream & liquid makeup is to apply in thin layers.

HOW TO APPLY CREAMS + LIQUIDS:

1. Put a little makeup on back of your hand.

2. Pick up makeup with dome blender brush.

3. Use dabbing & circular motions on back of hand to evenly distribute makeup into the bristles.

4. Apply color on paper with gentle swiping & circular motions.

5. Repeat steps 1-4 until you reach desired shade.

Eye Enhancements

• For a realistic eye color effect mix blue, green or orange eyeshadow with a bit of brown and/or grey eyeshadow. Fill in eye color with a pointed pencil brush.

• Add a coat of clear shiny nail polish over eye color for a natural glossy effect.

• Keep eraser handy to remove makeup that gets on whites of eyes.

Eyeliner Tips

• Apply a clear nail polish (matte or glossy top coat) over creamy eye pencils or liquid eyeliner to seal & keep from smudging.

• Substitute creamy eyeliner with products that dry and won't smudge. China Markers (by Dixon or Sharpie) make a great substitute for eye pencils. Fine-point permanent markers (by Sharpie) or ink (used with dip pen) can give you the look of rich liquid liner.

• Create the look of white eyeliner with liquid white-out corrector (look for it in a fine-point pen by BIC or Sharpie).

• Dark eyeshadow can be used in place of pencil & liquid eyeliners. For sharp crisp lines, apply with an angled liner brush. For a soft & smokey effect, line eyes with a pointed pencil brush.

Sparkle Effect

Glitter is a fun & easy way to add a touch of glitz & glam to your makeup looks.

HOW TO APPLY GLITTER:

1. Use brush or finger to spread an even layer of clear school or craft glue onto makeup chart (applying glue with tool will provide more even coverage).
2. Pour glitter over glue.
3. Hold makeup chart upright and tap to get rid of excess glitter. Be sure to lay paper under makeup chart to catch extra glitter.

Metallic Pigments

Highly-reflective metallic finishes are a great way to add a dimension and shine to makeup charts. For best results, use metallic pigments in powder form (eyeshadow, loose pigment, etc...). For application of liquid metallic makeup see tip on **'Cream + Liquid Makeup'**.

HOW TO APPLY METALLIC PIGMENTS:

1. Pick up powder on flat shader brush.
2. Lightly mist with water until slightly damp.
3. Distribute powder & water into the bristles by gently dabbing on the back of your hand.
4. Apply on paper with dabbing/pressing motions & let dry.
5. Use dry dome blender brush & metallic powder to blur any hard lines (use small circular motions along edges to create a seamless blend).

Cleaning Brushes

Using the same brush for multiple applications can easily lead to "muddy" colors. A simple way to avoid this is with a quick "dry cleaning" in between applications to remove color residue left on bristles. Simply wipe your brush on a damp baby wipe (or damp paper towel with a little baby shampoo lather). Then wipe bristles on a dry paper towel to remove excess moisture.

Adding Highlights

Highlights give face charts a pro look by adding dimension. Highlights can be easily achieved with the 'Reverse Highlighting Technique' - simply add color to makeup chart then use an eraser to remove color where you want highlights to be.

Lip Color

• Substitute creamy lip products with powder eyeshadow or colored pencils.

• Real lipgloss is not recommended for makeup charts as it can easily smear. A great substitute for lip gloss is shiny clear nail polish. Apply a coat of clear shiny nail polish over lips for glossy effect.

• Create your own custom tinted "lipgloss" by mixing clear nail polish & powder eyeshadow.

• To create a tinted gloss in a shade similar to real lips, mix clear nail polish with peachy-mauve eyeshadow or blush. Add matte white eyeshadow to lighten and make more opaque.

HOW TO MAKE TINTED LIPGLOSS:

1. Cut a square piece of foil (about 4 x 4 inches). Gently push a finger into the center of foil to create a bowl.

2. Pour clear nail polish in bowl until 1/4 - 1/2 full.

3. Scrap a little bit of eyeshadow into bowl using needle or toothpick.

4. Mix powder & polish well with applicator brush.

5. Test color on white piece of scrap paper. Keep adding eyeshadow & testing until you reach desired shade. If color is too dark, add more clear polish or white eyeshadow.

6. Apply color to lips immediatley.
Clean applicator brush with nail polish remover before dipping back into polish bottle.

Set and Seal

Protect & preserve completed face charts from moisture, fading and smearing with an 'artist fixative' or 'paper protectant' spray. You will need a well-ventilated area when using these types of products - please follow directions carefully!
*Krylon Preserve It Matte' is recommended.

how-to tutorial
HIGHLIGHT + CONTOUR

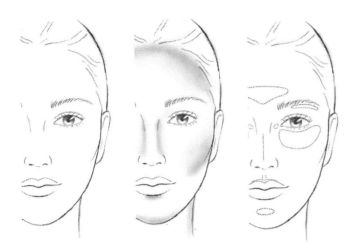

WHAT YOU NEED
....

Brushes
☐ Dome blender
☐ Flat shader
☐ Pointed pencil

Makeup
☐ Mid-tone
☐ Contour
☐ Highlight
☐ Mid-tone

The purpose of highlighting & contouring is to enhance & define the natural structure of a face. Its done by adding strategic placement of light and shadows. Adding light creates the illusion of features coming forward while adding shadow (contour) creates the illusion of features drawing back.

Makeup artists often choose to highlight & contour their face charts to achieve a realistic dimensional look. Although there are some differences in application when it comes to a facechart vs. a real face, the overall effect is similar.

This tutorial is intended to teach you the basics of highlighting & contouring to define a female and male face. Practice face charts are included in this book to help you build your skills!

OTHER WAYS TO USE HIGHLIGHT + CONTOUR

Hightlight & contour can also used to "sculpt & shape" the natural facial structure for extra enhancement & corrective purposes. Examples include:

- Minimize unfavorable features (chubby cheeks, wide forehead)
- Elongate wide features (lengthen round or square face)
- Soften strong features (round out angular jaw, chin, hairline)
- Balance uneven facial structure

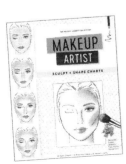

If your interested in learning advanced corrective techniques, be sure to check out 'Sculpt & Shape Charts' from The Beauty Studio Collection.

The book contains a indepth step-by-step guide along with 7 face shapes to practice on!

Look for it on coloristabooks.com

HOW TO CHOOSE SHADES

Mid-tone

Decided on a flesh-toned skincolor and choose a matching face powder.

Highlight
Choose a flesh-tone powder 2-3 shades lighter than the skincolor (or instead use white of paper as highlight).

Contour
Choose a bronzer or contour powder 2-3 shades darker than the skincolor.

Blush
Choose a neutral rosy blush shade. You can create your own by mixing pink blush with skintoned face power.

Female Face
HIGHLIGHT + CONTOUR GUIDE

An **Oval** face is considered to be the "ideal" or "perfect" shape because it's portionally balanced. The highlight & contour method for an oval face focuses on defining the natural facial structure.

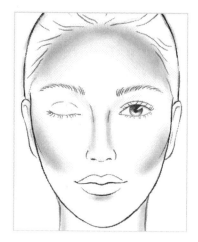

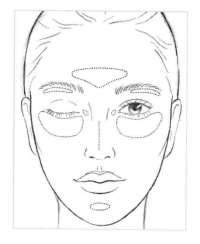

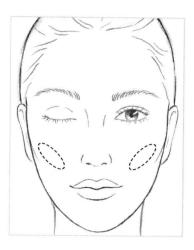

STEP 1: CONTOUR

Contour is applied on the natural recesses of the face. Use dome blender brush & contour powder to softly shade:

Hairline
Under cheekbones (curved line)
Sides of neck (optional)

Define shading along **hairline & under cheekbones** with flat shader brush & contour powder.

Add shading to **sides of nose & under bottom lip** with pencil brush & contour powder.

STEP 2: HIGHLIGHT + MID-TONE

Highlights are placed on the high points of the face. Use dome blender brush to apply highlight powder to (or leave areas blank if using white of paper as highlight):

Forehead
Browbone
Inner eye corners
Under eyes
Cheekbones
Bridge of nose
Cupids bow
Center of chin

Apply mid-tone skincolor to blank areas between contour & highlight. Use small circular motions to create a seamless blend.

STEP 3: BLUSH

For added shape & natural flush of color, use blender brush to apply blush color in an upward diagnol oval on apples of cheek.

TIP *When it comes to applying blush on a real female face, general rule of thumb is to stop below center of eye or at least a finger width distance from nose.*

PRO TIPS

When contouring cheekbones on a face chart, follow an imaginary line from the MIDDLE of the ear to the CORNER of the lip - STOP when you reach center of eye.

When contouring cheekbones on a real face, follow an imaginary line from the TOP of the ear to the CORNER of the lip - STOP when you reach center of eye. Add extra definition to a real face by shading along & under jawline. Slim & minimize a double chin by contouring under chin downwards towards neck.

Male Face

HIGHLIGHT + CONTOUR GUIDE

The masculine highlight and contour method on a **Male** face focuses on defining the strong angular structure.

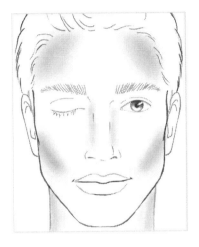

STEP 1: CONTOUR

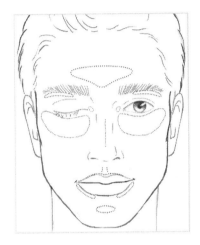

STEP 2: HIGHLIGHT + MID-TONE

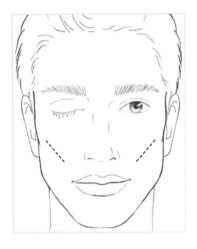

STEP 3: BLUSH

STEP 1: CONTOUR

Contour is applied on the natural recesses of the face. Use dome blender brush & contour powder to softly shade:

Sides of forehead
Under cheekbones (straight line)
Sides of neck (optional)

Define shading along **sides of forehead & under cheekbones** with flat shader brush & contour powder.

Add shading to **sides of nose** with pencil brush & contour powder.

STEP 2: HIGHLIGHT + MID-TONE

Highlights are placed on the high points of the face. Use dome blender brush to apply highlight powder to (or leave areas blank if using white of paper as highlight)::

Forehead
Browbone
Inner eye corners
Under eyes
Cheekbones
Bridge of nose
Cupids bow
Center of chin

Apply mid-tone skincolor to blank areas between contour & highlight. Use small circular motions to create a seamless blend.

STEP 3: BLUSH

Strengthen sharpness of jawline by adding blush following the same angle as cheekbone contour.

TIP Use light hand when applying blush. If blush looks to bright, dull it down by blending skintone powder over it.

DRAWING EYELASHES

A full set of lashes is a fab way to customize your makeup charts. When it comes to drawing lashes, you'll want to use a drawing tool that's opaque, adheres to paper over makeup & is fine enough to create delicate lash "hairs" with.

Liquid eyeliner, sharpie markers & dark color pencils are common drawing tools but can sometimes be challenging to work with because they either aren't fine enough to draw fine lash strokes with or don't show up very good over eyeshadow.

A far better option, although a little untraditional, is ink & a dip pen. India/Sumi ink is thin yet opaque & permanent when dry. When used together with a dip pen & a fine-nib, you can create thick to thin hair-like strokes with smooth precision. Speedball offers inexpensive ink & dip pen sets (Sketching or Mapping Project Set is recommended).

In this tutorial you will learn how to draw 4 styles of lashes. Each style varies in density giving your a range of looks from light to ultra full & dramatic. But before we jump into drawing full sets of lashes, it's helpful to begin with the basics. 'Drawing Lashes 101' will guide you on drawing individual "lash hairs".

Eyelash Styles

Natural   *Wispy*

Glamour   *Bombshell*

DRAWING LASHES 101

WHAT YOU NEED   ☐ Drawing tool ☐ Scrap paper ☐ Eye practice chart

STEP 1: PREP DRAWING TOOL

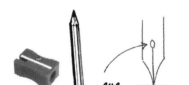

Pencil user: Sharpen pencil so that you can create fine strokes (lines) that mimic natural lash hairs. Keep sharpener handy as point can quickly become dull when drawing.

Dip pen + ink user: Dip nib into ink just past the eye. Scribble on scrap paper to remove excess ink.

Please note: Dried up ink on nibs can be difficult to remove & block ink flow. After every drawing session, it's recommended to clean nibs with window cleaner & an old soft toothbrush. Dry thoroughly with cloth or paper towel to prevent from rusting.

STEP 2: PRACTICE STROKE

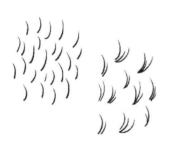

A stroke is a line that reduces in thickness towards one end. Real eyelashes resemble curved tapered strokes. To create tapered strokes, press down drawing tool with some pressure begin reducing pressure as you draw a small curved line. On a scrap piece of paper, practice single strokes & clusters of 2-3 strokes (of varying lengths).

STEP 3: PRACTICE STROKE DIRECTION

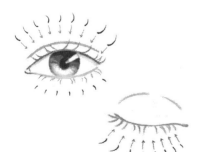

Open Eye: Starting at inner part of eye draw short strokes (in the same direction as the letter "C") until you reach the iris. At the iris begin drawing strokes the direction as a backwards letter "C". Increase length & tilt of strokes as you move towards outer corner. For bottom lashes, mirror top lashes using shorter strokes.

Closed Eye: Starting at inner part of eye draw short strokes (in the same direction as a backwards letter "C"). Increase length & tilt of stroke as you move along eye towards outer corner.

DRAWING LASH STYLES

WHAT YOU NEED ☐ Drawing tool ☐ Eye or face chart

Note: Lash strokes were drawn above the eye to provide you with a clear view of the strokes drawn on the lashline.

HOW TO DRAW
Natural Lash Style

1. Draw 1st set of lashes for open & closed eye.

2. Add a few single lashes between gaps.

3. Continue adding single lashes & a few clusters to add fullness. For the most natural look do not fill in all gaps - you should be able to see the eyelid through the lashes.

4. Draw bottom lashes on open eye (optional).

HOW TO DRAW
Wispy Lash Style

1. Draw 1st set of lashes for open & closed eye (draw mostly clusters of varying lengths).

2. Add a few single lashes & clusters of varying lengths between gaps.

3. Continue adding single lashes & clusters. For natural results do not fill in all gaps - you should be able to see the some of the eyelid through the lashes.

4. Draw bottom lashes on open eye (optional).

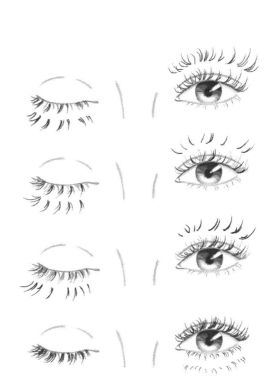

HOW TO DRAW
Bombshell Lash Style

1. Draw 1st set of lashes for open & closed eye. Draw short, med and long clusters. Start with shortest ones near inner corner, med towards center and longest near outer corner.

2. Add a few single lashes and clusters of varying lengths between gaps.

3. Continue adding single lashes & clusters of varying lengths. For the most natural look fill in most gaps (but not all) to create the illusion of fullness.

4. Draw bottom lashes on open eye (optional).

HOW TO DRAW
Glamour Lash Style

1. Draw 1st set of lashes for open & closed eye draw mainly thick clusters of varying lengths).

2. Add a single lashes & clusters of varying lengths between gaps.

3. Continue adding single lashes & clusters of varing lengths to increase density (fill in the majority of gaps-you shouldn't be able to see much of the eyelid through the lashes).

4. Draw bottom lashes on open eye (optional).

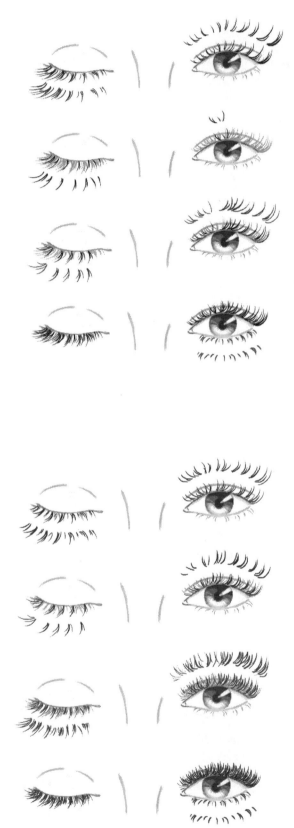

how-to tutorial
DRAWING EYEBROWS

Similarly to lashes, brows can play a important role in a makeup look. Although are many styles of brows, they can be simplified down to 5 shapes of varying thickness: Straight, Round, Soft angle, Sharp Angle & S-shape.

When it comes to drawing brows on paper, you'll want to choose a drawing tool that allows you to create hair-like strokes with precision. You'll find that lead/colored pencils or thin markers work best for brows as they offer a fine point, come in natural brow shades and won't smudge like creamy eye/brow pencils do.

It's important to note that drawing brows involves erasing, so you may want to consider applying eye or face after brows application (this will eliminate having to reapply makeup that you accidently removed/erased).

To get started, follow 'Brow Drawing Basics' to become familiar with drawing realistic brow hairs. When you are ready to draw your own custom brows, follow 'How to Draw Brows from Scratch'.

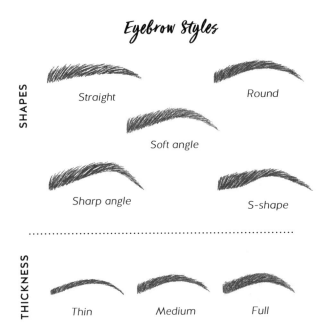

Eyebrow Styles

SHAPES

Straight   Round

Soft angle

Sharp angle   S-shape

THICKNESS

Thin   Medium   Full

BROW DRAWING BASICS

WHAT YOU NEED   ☐ Pencil (lead or colored) ☐ Sharpener ☐ Scrap paper
☐ Eye or brow chart

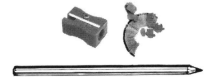

STEP 1: PREP TOOL

Sharpen pencil so that you can create fine strokes (lines) that mimic natural brow hairs. Keep sharpener handy as point can quickly become dull when drawing.

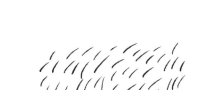

STEP 2: PRACTICE STROKES

A stroke is a line that reduces in thickness towards on end. Real brow hairs resemble curved tapered strokes. Brow hairs generally grow straight up at the inner part of the brow and then begin to tilt outwards.

On a scrap peice of paper, practice single strokes of varying lengths. To create a tapered stroke, press pencil down with some pressure - begin reducing pressure as you draw a small curved line.

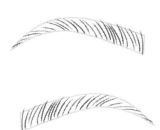

STEP 3: PRACTICE STROKE DIRECTION

Fill in pre-outlined brow with hair strokes:

LEFT BROW: Start at inner part of brow, draw a few vertical strokes then start tilting strokes outwards to the LEFT - when you reach the highest point of the arch shorten length of strokes.

RIGHT BROW: Start at inner part of brow, draw a few vertical strokes then start tilting strokes outwards to the RIGHT - when you reach the highest point of the arch shorten length of strokes.

DRAWING BROWS FROM SCRATCH

WHAT YOU NEED

☐ Ruler ☐ Pencil ☐ Eraser ☐ Pencil brush ☐ Brow powder
☐ Colored pencil (in brow shade of choice)

PART ONE

Mapping Brows

Follow the 3 point method to determine where a brow starts, highest point of arch & where it ends. Use a ruler & pencil to lightly mark points. When mapping brows, consider the space between the lid & brows. Higher placement offers more space for eyeshadow but can also create a permanently surprised look.

A. Beginning of brow aligns with center of nostril.

B. Highest point of arch aligns with edge of nostril and center of iris (on closed eye measure to approximately center of eye).

C. End of brow aligns with edge of nostril & the outer corner of eye.

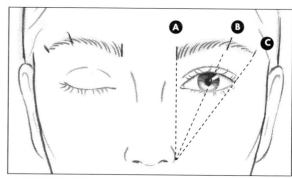

  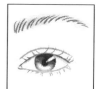

Example of low, medium & high brow placement

PART TWO

Outline + Fill

1. After mapping brows, use pencil to lightly sketch an outline of the brow shape. Keep eraser handy to make corrections as needed.

2. With a colored pencil, fill in shape with hairlike strokes. Start at beginning with a few vertical strokes then fill in rest of shape with tilted strokes.*

3. Lightly erase pencil marks & brow outline.

4. Fill in sparse areas with brow powder & pencil brush.

5. Use colored pencil to redefine strokes. Add more strokes of various lengths in sparse areas for extra dimension & definition.

6. Use eraser lightly around edges of brows to clean up any smudges and further define shape. Touch up and/or add more hairstrokes in sparse areas (optional).

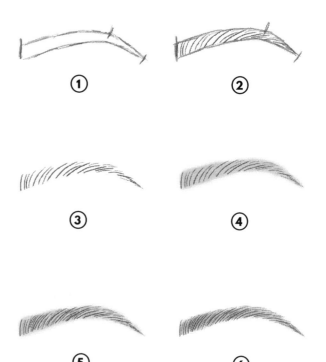

 PRO TIPS

If you have trouble sketching brow shape outline freehand, try using a brow stencil.

Steps 4-6 can be used to further enhance pre-drawn or pre-outlined brows that have been filled in with brow hairs.

how-to tutorial
PRO LIP EFFECTS

Nude Lips

WHAT YOU NEED
☐ Pencil brush ☐ Nude lipcolor
☐ Lipliner ☐ Eraser

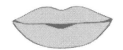 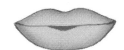

1. Apply nude color to entire lips with pencil brush.

2. Apply liner to outer edge of lips with pencil brush. Use small circular motions where dark & light meet to create a seamless blend.

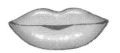 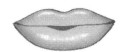

3. Use eraser to add highlights on upper & bottom lip.

4. Optional: Apply coat of shiny clear polish for a glossy finish.

Ombre Lips

WHAT YOU NEED
☐ Pencil brush ☐ Angled liner brush
☐ Light lipcolor ☐ Dark lipcolor

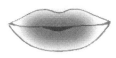 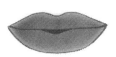

1. Apply lightest color to center of lips with pencil brush (concentrate the most color in the center & gradually fade out.)

2. Apply darkest color on outer edges of lips with pencil brush. Use small circular motions where dark meets light to create a seamless blend.

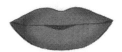 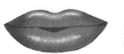

3. Add more dark color to intensify outer edges of lips. Apply with angled liner brush - use soft strokes to avoid harsh lines.

4. Optional: For a glossy ombre, use eraser to add highlights & apply coat of shiny clear polish.

PRO TIPS

- See 'Pro Tips + Tricks' for how-to on mixing your own tinted lipgloss.
- When using light nude shades on dark skintones, use a brown lip liner to create a seamless transition from skin to lips.
- If a nude lip is too pale, tone it down with tinted lipgloss in a shade similar to natural lips (neutral peachy-mauve).

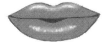

Glossy Lips

For full plump lips with a high-shine finish.

WHAT YOU NEED:
Lip color, pencil brush, eraser, clear shiny nail polish

HOW TO APPLY:
1. Color in lips with pencil brush.
2. Add reflection on upper & bottom lip with eraser.
3. Apply a coat of polish for a glossy finish.

Ombre Lips

Achieve rich velvety texture without the mess of matte liquid lipstick.

WHAT YOU NEED:
Marker (choice of lipcolor) matte eyeshadow (same shade as lipcolor), pencil brush

HOW TO APPLY:
1. Fill in lips with marker
2. Use pencil brush to apply matte eyeshadow over marker.

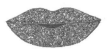

Glitter Lips

Add a touch of glitz & glam to your looks with sparkle.

WHAT YOU NEED:
Glitter, clear school glue*, finger or brush to apply glue, clear shiny nail polish

HOW TO APPLY:
1. Spread thin layer of glue on lips.
2. Pour glitter on lips.
3. Remove excess glitter.
4. Seal glitter with coat of polish.

* Clear glue works best with glitter as white glue can dry cloudy & dull shine.

EYE PRACTICE CHARTS

Use templates to design looks and practice application techniques.

_____

_____

_____

_____

_____

_____

_____

_____

_____

_____

_____

_____

_____

_____

_____

_____

_____

_____

_____

EYE PRACTICE CHARTS

Use templates to design looks and practice application techniques.

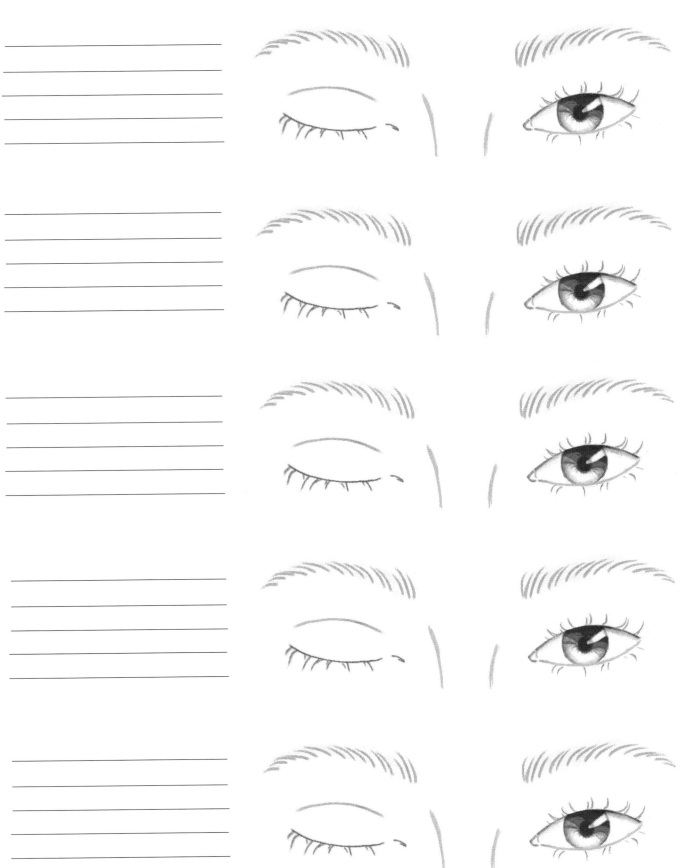

EYE PRACTICE CHARTS

Use templates to design looks and practice application techniques.

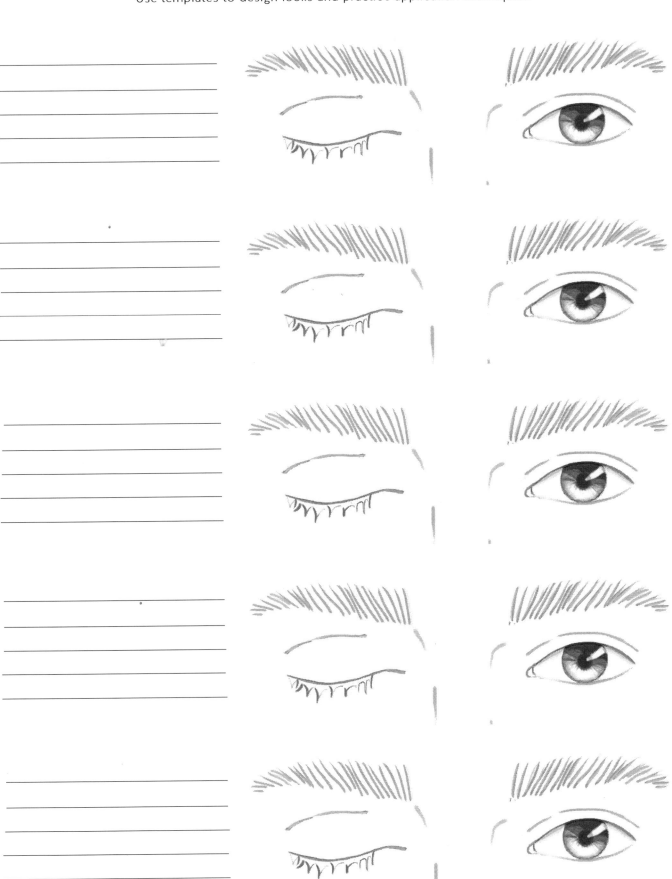

LIP PRACTICE CHARTS

Use templates to design looks and practice application techniques.

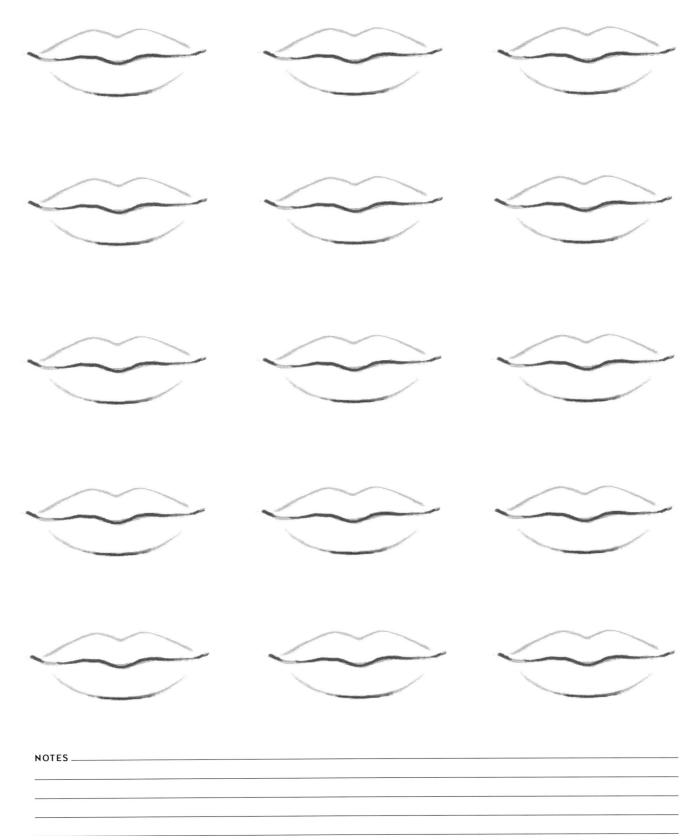

NOTES _____

_____

_____

_____

_____

BROW PRACTICE CHARTS

Use templates to fill in pre-outlined brow shapes

NOTES

Straight

Round

Soft Angle

Sharp Angle

S-shape

BLANK BROW
PRACTICE CHARTS

Use templates to draw brows from scratch by mapping, outlining shape and filliing in.

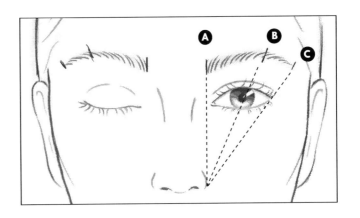

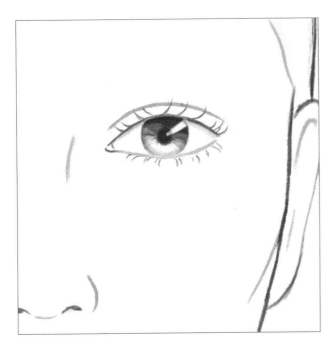

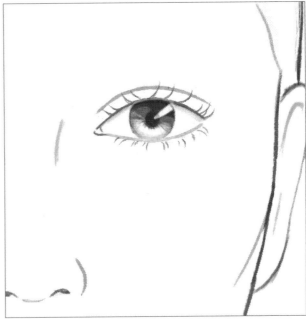

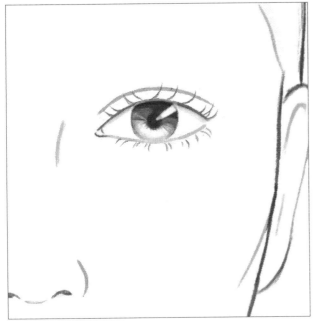

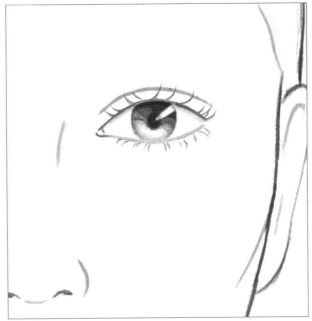

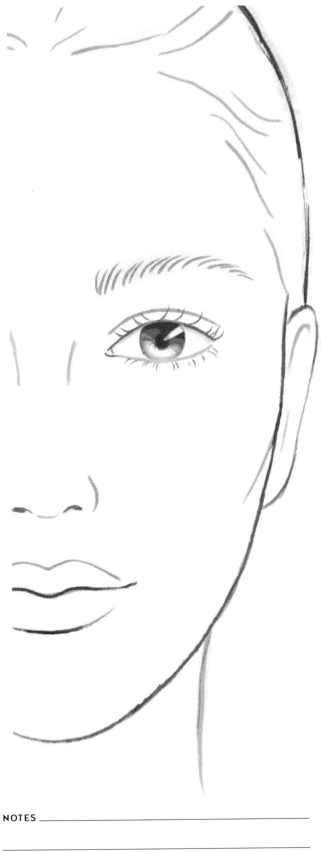

NOTES _____

_____

_____

_____

NOTES _____

_____

_____

_____

BRUSHES + TOOLS

_____

_____

_____

_____

NOTES

_____

_____

_____

_____

_____

_____

BRUSHES + TOOLS

_____

_____

_____

_____

NOTES

_____

_____

_____

_____

_____

_____

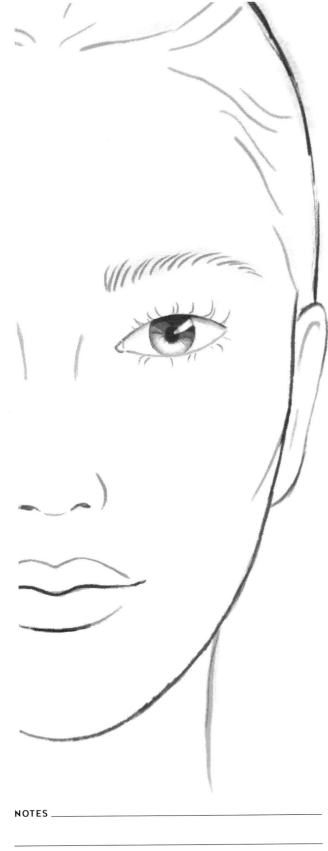

NOTES _____
_____
_____
_____
_____

NOTES _____
_____
_____
_____
_____

BRUSHES + TOOLS

_____

_____

_____

_____

NOTES

_____

_____

_____

_____

_____

_____

BRUSHES + TOOLS

_____

_____

_____

_____

NOTES

_____

_____

_____

_____

_____

_____

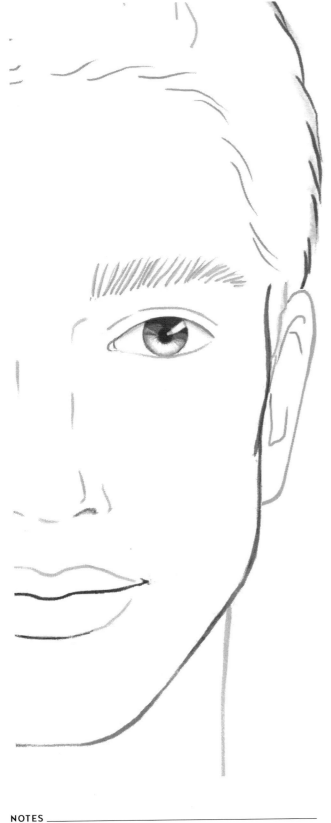

NOTES _____

_____

_____

_____

_____

NOTES _____

_____

_____

_____

_____

BRUSHES + TOOLS

_____

_____

_____

_____

NOTES

_____

_____

_____

_____

_____

_____

BRUSHES + TOOLS

_____

_____

_____

_____

NOTES

_____

_____

_____

_____

_____

makeup face chart

LOOK NAME

_____

EYES

Brows:_____

Base:_____

Eye shadow:_____

_____

_____

Eyeliner:_____

Mascara:_____

Lashes:_____

FACE

Primer: _____

Concealer: _____

Foundation:_____

Powder:_____

Blush: _____

Bronzer: _____

Contour: _____

Highlight:_____

LIPS

Liner:_____

Gloss:_____

Color:_____

_____

CLIENT NAME

_____

MAKEUP ARTIST

_____

BRUSHES + TOOLS

_____

_____

_____

_____

_____

NOTES

_____

_____

_____

_____

_____

makeup face chart

LOOK NAME

_____

EYES

Brows:_____

Base:_____

Eye shadow:_____

_____

Eyeliner:_____

Mascara:_____

Lashes:_____

FACE

Primer: _____

Concealer: _____

Foundation: _____

Powder:_____

Blush: _____

Bronzer: _____

Contour: _____

Highlight:_____

LIPS

Liner:_____

Gloss:_____

Color:_____

_____

CLIENT NAME

_____

MAKEUP ARTIST

_____

makeup face chart

LOOK NAME

_____

EYES

Brows:_____

Base:_____

Eye shadow:_____

_____

_____

Eyeliner:_____

Mascara:_____

Lashes:_____

FACE

Primer: _____

Concealer: _____

Foundation: _____

Powder: _____

Blush: _____

Bronzer: _____

Contour: _____

Highlight: _____

LIPS

Liner:_____

Gloss:_____

Color:_____

_____

CLIENT NAME

_____

MAKEUP ARTIST

_____

BRUSHES + TOOLS

_____

_____

_____

_____

_____

NOTES

_____

_____

_____

_____

_____

makeup face chart

LOOK NAME

_____

EYES

Brows:_____

Base:_____

Eye shadow:_____

_____

_____

Eyeliner:_____

Mascara:_____

Lashes:_____

FACE

Primer: _____

Concealer:_____

Foundation:_____

Powder:_____

Blush:_____

Bronzer:_____

Contour:_____

Highlight:_____

LIPS

Liner:_____

Gloss:_____

Color:_____

_____

CLIENT NAME

_____

MAKEUP ARTIST

_____

BRUSHES + TOOLS

_____

_____

_____

_____

_____

NOTES

_____

_____

_____

_____

_____

makeup face chart

LOOK NAME

_____

EYES

Brows:_____

Base:_____

Eye shadow:_____

_____

Eyeliner:_____

Mascara:_____

Lashes:_____

FACE

Primer: _____

Concealer: _____

Foundation: _____

Powder: _____

Blush: _____

Bronzer: _____

Contour: _____

Highlight: _____

LIPS

Liner:_____

Gloss:_____

Color:_____

_____

CLIENT NAME

_____

MAKEUP ARTIST

_____

makeup face chart

LOOK NAME

_____

EYES

Brows:_____

Base:_____

Eye shadow:_____

_____

_____

Eyeliner:_____

Mascara:_____

Lashes:_____

FACE

Primer: _____

Concealer: _____

Foundation: _____

Powder:_____

Blush: _____

Bronzer: _____

Contour: _____

Highlight:_____

LIPS

Liner:_____

Gloss:_____

Color:_____

_____

CLIENT NAME

_____

MAKEUP ARTIST

_____

BRUSHES + TOOLS

_____

_____

_____

_____

_____

NOTES

_____

_____

_____

_____

_____

makeup face chart

LOOK NAME

_____

EYES

Brows:_____

Base:_____

Eye shadow:_____

_____

Eyeliner:_____

Mascara:_____

Lashes:_____

FACE

Primer: _____

Concealer:_____

Foundation:_____

Powder:_____

Blush:_____

Bronzer:_____

Contour:_____

Highlight:_____

LIPS

Liner:_____

Gloss:_____

Color:_____

_____

CLIENT NAME

_____

MAKEUP ARTIST

_____

BRUSHES + TOOLS

_____

_____

_____

_____

_____

NOTES

_____

_____

_____

_____

_____

makeup face chart

LOOK NAME

_____

EYES

Brows:_____

Base:_____

Eye shadow:_____

_____

_____

Eyeliner:_____

Mascara:_____

Lashes:_____

FACE

Primer: _____

Concealer: _____

Foundation:_____

Powder:_____

Blush:_____

Bronzer:_____

Contour:_____

Highlight:_____

LIPS

Liner:_____

Gloss:_____

Color:_____

_____

CLIENT NAME

_____

MAKEUP ARTIST

_____

BRUSHES + TOOLS

_____

_____

_____

_____

_____

NOTES

_____

_____

_____

_____

_____

makeup face chart

LOOK NAME

_____

EYES

Brows:_____

Base:_____

Eye shadow:_____

_____

Eyeliner:_____

Mascara:_____

Lashes:_____

FACE

Primer: _____

Concealer:_____

Foundation:_____

Powder:_____

Blush:_____

Bronzer:_____

Contour:_____

Highlight:_____

LIPS

Liner:_____

Gloss:_____

Color:_____

_____

CLIENT NAME

_____

MAKEUP ARTIST

_____

BRUSHES + TOOLS

_____

_____

_____

_____

_____

NOTES

_____

_____

_____

_____

_____

makeup face chart

LOOK NAME

_____

EYES

Brows:_____

Base:_____

Eye shadow:_____

_____

Eyeliner:_____

Mascara:_____

Lashes:_____

FACE

Primer: _____

Concealer: _____

Foundation: _____

Powder:_____

Blush: _____

Bronzer: _____

Contour: _____

Highlight:_____

LIPS

Liner:_____

Gloss:_____

Color:_____

_____

CLIENT NAME

_____

MAKEUP ARTIST

_____

makeup face chart

LOOK NAME

_____

EYES

Brows:_____

Base:_____

Eye shadow:_____

_____

_____

Eyeliner:_____

Mascara:_____

Lashes:_____

FACE

Primer: _____

Concealer: _____

Foundation: _____

Powder:_____

Blush: _____

Bronzer: _____

Contour: _____

Highlight:_____

LIPS

Liner:_____

Gloss:_____

Color:_____

_____

CLIENT NAME

_____

MAKEUP ARTIST

_____

BRUSHES + TOOLS

NOTES

makeup face chart

LOOK NAME

_____

EYES

Brows:_____

Base:_____

Eye shadow:_____

_____

_____

Eyeliner:_____

Mascara:_____

Lashes:_____

FACE

Primer: _____

Concealer: _____

Foundation:_____

Powder:_____

Blush:_____

Bronzer: _____

Contour:_____

Highlight:_____

LIPS

Liner:_____

Gloss:_____

Color:_____

_____

CLIENT NAME

_____

MAKEUP ARTIST

_____

BRUSHES + TOOLS

_____

_____

_____

_____

_____

NOTES

_____

_____

_____

_____

_____

makeup face chart

LOOK NAME

_____

EYES

Brows:_____

Base:_____

Eye shadow:_____

_____

_____

Eyeliner:_____

Mascara:_____

Lashes:_____

FACE

Primer: _____

Concealer: _____

Foundation: _____

Powder:_____

Blush: _____

Bronzer:_____

Contour:_____

Highlight:_____

LIPS

Liner:_____

Gloss:_____

Color:_____

_____

CLIENT NAME

_____

MAKEUP ARTIST

_____

BRUSHES + TOOLS

_____

_____

_____

_____

_____

NOTES

_____

_____

_____

_____

_____

makeup face chart

LOOK NAME

_____

EYES

Brows:_____

Base:_____

Eye shadow:_____

_____

Eyeliner:_____

Mascara:_____

Lashes:_____

FACE

Primer: _____

Concealer: _____

Foundation:_____

Powder:_____

Blush: _____

Bronzer: _____

Contour: _____

Highlight:_____

LIPS

Liner:_____

Gloss:_____

Color:_____

_____

CLIENT NAME

_____

MAKEUP ARTIST

_____

63

BRUSHES + TOOLS

_____

_____

_____

_____

_____

NOTES

_____

_____

_____

_____

_____

makeup face chart

LOOK NAME

_____

EYES

Brows:_____

Base:_____

Eye shadow:_____

_____

Eyeliner:_____

Mascara:_____

Lashes:_____

FACE

Primer: _____

Concealer:_____

Foundation:_____

Powder:_____

Blush:_____

Bronzer:_____

Contour:_____

Highlight:_____

LIPS

Liner:_____

Gloss:_____

Color:_____

_____

CLIENT NAME

_____

MAKEUP ARTIST

_____

makeup face chart

LOOK NAME

_____

EYES

Brows:_____

Base:_____

Eye shadow:_____

_____

Eyeliner:_____

Mascara:_____

Lashes:_____

FACE

Primer: _____

Concealer: _____

Foundation:_____

Powder:_____

Blush: _____

Bronzer: _____

Contour: _____

Highlight:_____

LIPS

Liner:_____

Gloss:_____

Color:_____

_____

CLIENT NAME

_____

MAKEUP ARTIST

_____

67

BRUSHES + TOOLS

_____

_____

_____

_____

_____

NOTES

_____

_____

_____

_____

_____

makeup face chart

LOOK NAME

_____

EYES

Brows:_____

Base:_____

Eye shadow:_____

_____

_____

Eyeliner:_____

Mascara:_____

Lashes:_____

FACE

Primer: _____

Concealer: _____

Foundation:_____

Powder:_____

Blush: _____

Bronzer:_____

Contour:_____

Highlight:_____

LIPS

Liner:_____

Gloss:_____

Color:_____

_____

CLIENT NAME

_____

MAKEUP ARTIST

_____

makeup face chart

LOOK NAME

_____

EYES

Brows:_____

Base:_____

Eye shadow:_____

_____

_____

Eyeliner:_____

Mascara:_____

Lashes:_____

FACE

Primer: _____

Concealer: _____

Foundation: _____

Powder:_____

Blush: _____

Bronzer: _____

Contour: _____

Highlight:_____

LIPS

Liner:_____

Gloss:_____

Color:_____

_____

CLIENT NAME

_____

MAKEUP ARTIST

_____

BRUSHES + TOOLS

_____

_____

_____

_____

_____

NOTES

_____

_____

_____

_____

_____

makeup face chart

LOOK NAME

_____

EYES

Brows:_____

Base:_____

Eye shadow:_____

_____

_____

Eyeliner:_____

Mascara:_____

Lashes:_____

FACE

Primer: _____

Concealer: _____

Foundation: _____

Powder:_____

Blush: _____

Bronzer: _____

Contour: _____

Highlight:_____

LIPS

Liner:_____

Gloss:_____

Color:_____

_____

CLIENT NAME

_____

MAKEUP ARTIST

_____

BRUSHES + TOOLS

_____

_____

_____

_____

_____

NOTES

_____

_____

_____

_____

_____

makeup face chart

LOOK NAME

_____

EYES

Brows:_____

Base:_____

Eye shadow:_____

_____

_____

Eyeliner:_____

Mascara:_____

Lashes:_____

FACE

Primer: _____

Concealer: _____

Foundation:_____

Powder:_____

Blush: _____

Bronzer:_____

Contour:_____

Highlight:_____

LIPS

Liner:_____

Gloss:_____

Color:_____

_____

CLIENT NAME

_____

MAKEUP ARTIST

_____

75

BRUSHES + TOOLS

_____

_____

_____

_____

_____

NOTES

_____

_____

_____

_____

_____

makeup face chart

LOOK NAME

_____

EYES

Brows:_____

Base:_____

Eye shadow:_____

_____

_____

Eyeliner:_____

Mascara:_____

Lashes:_____

FACE

Primer: _____

Concealer: _____

Foundation: _____

Powder:_____

Blush: _____

Bronzer: _____

Contour: _____

Highlight:_____

LIPS

Liner:_____

Gloss:_____

Color:_____

_____

CLIENT NAME

_____

MAKEUP ARTIST

_____

BRUSHES + TOOLS

_____

_____

_____

_____

_____

NOTES

_____

_____

_____

_____

_____

makeup face chart

LOOK NAME

_____

EYES

Brows:_____

Base:_____

Eye shadow:_____

_____

_____

Eyeliner:_____

Mascara:_____

Lashes:_____

FACE

Primer: _____

Concealer: _____

Foundation: _____

Powder: _____

Blush: _____

Bronzer: _____

Contour: _____

Highlight: _____

LIPS

Liner:_____

Gloss:_____

Color:_____

_____

CLIENT NAME

_____

MAKEUP ARTIST

_____

BRUSHES + TOOLS

_____

_____

_____

_____

_____

NOTES

_____

_____

_____

_____

_____

makeup face chart

LOOK NAME

_____

EYES

Brows:_____

Base:_____

Eye shadow:_____

_____

_____

Eyeliner:_____

Mascara:_____

Lashes:_____

FACE

Primer: _____

Concealer: _____

Foundation: _____

Powder:_____

Blush: _____

Bronzer: _____

Contour: _____

Highlight:_____

LIPS

Liner:_____

Gloss:_____

Color:_____

_____

CLIENT NAME

_____

MAKEUP ARTIST

_____

makeup face chart

LOOK NAME

_____

EYES

Brows:_____

Base:_____

Eye shadow:_____

_____

_____

Eyeliner:_____

Mascara:_____

Lashes:_____

FACE

Primer: _____

Concealer: _____

Foundation:_____

Powder:_____

Blush: _____

Bronzer:_____

Contour:_____

Highlight:_____

LIPS

Liner:_____

Gloss:_____

Color:_____

_____

CLIENT NAME

_____

MAKEUP ARTIST

_____

BRUSHES + TOOLS

_____

_____

_____

_____

_____

NOTES

_____

_____

_____

_____

_____

makeup face chart

LOOK NAME

_____

EYES

Brows:_____

Base:_____

Eye shadow:_____

_____

_____

Eyeliner:_____

Mascara:_____

Lashes:_____

FACE

Primer: _____

Concealer: _____

Foundation:_____

Powder:_____

Blush: _____

Bronzer: _____

Contour: _____

Highlight:_____

LIPS

Liner:_____

Gloss:_____

Color:_____

_____

CLIENT NAME

_____

MAKEUP ARTIST

_____

makeup face chart

LOOK NAME
_____

EYES

Brows:_____

Base:_____

Eye shadow:_____

_____

_____

Eyeliner:_____

Mascara:_____

Lashes:_____

FACE

Primer: _____

Concealer:_____

Foundation:_____

Powder:_____

Blush:_____

Bronzer:_____

Contour:_____

Highlight:_____

LIPS

Liner:_____

Gloss:_____

Color:_____

_____

CLIENT NAME
_____

MAKEUP ARTIST
_____

BRUSHES + TOOLS

_____

_____

_____

_____

_____

NOTES

_____

_____

_____

_____

_____

makeup face chart

LOOK NAME

_____

EYES

Brows:_____

Base:_____

Eye shadow:_____

_____

_____

Eyeliner:_____

Mascara:_____

Lashes:_____

FACE

Primer: _____

Concealer: _____

Foundation:_____

Powder:_____

Blush: _____

Bronzer: _____

Contour: _____

Highlight:_____

LIPS

Liner:_____

Gloss:_____

Color:_____

_____

CLIENT NAME

_____

MAKEUP ARTIST

_____

89

makeup face chart

LOOK NAME

_____

EYES

Brows:_____

Base:_____

Eye shadow:_____

_____

_____

Eyeliner:_____

Mascara:_____

Lashes:_____

FACE

Primer: _____

Concealer: _____

Foundation: _____

Powder:_____

Blush: _____

Bronzer: _____

Contour: _____

Highlight:_____

LIPS

Liner:_____

Gloss:_____

Color:_____

_____

CLIENT NAME

_____

MAKEUP ARTIST

_____

makeup face chart

LOOK NAME

_____

EYES

Brows:_____

Base:_____

Eye shadow:_____

_____

_____

Eyeliner:_____

Mascara:_____

Lashes:_____

FACE

Primer: _____

Concealer: _____

Foundation:_____

Powder:_____

Blush: _____

Bronzer: _____

Contour: _____

Highlight:_____

LIPS

Liner:_____

Gloss:_____

Color:_____

_____

CLIENT NAME

_____

MAKEUP ARTIST

_____

BRUSHES + TOOLS

_____

_____

_____

_____

_____

NOTES

_____

_____

_____

_____

_____

makeup face chart

LOOK NAME

_____

EYES

Brows:_____

Base:_____

Eye shadow:_____

_____

_____

Eyeliner:_____

Mascara:_____

Lashes:_____

FACE

Primer: _____

Concealer:_____

Foundation:_____

Powder:_____

Blush:_____

Bronzer:_____

Contour:_____

Highlight:_____

LIPS

Liner:_____

Gloss:_____

Color:_____

_____

CLIENT NAME

_____

MAKEUP ARTIST

_____

makeup face chart

LOOK NAME

_____

EYES

Brows:_____

Base:_____

Eye shadow:_____

_____

_____

Eyeliner:_____

Mascara:_____

Lashes:_____

FACE

Primer: _____

Concealer:_____

Foundation:_____

Powder:_____

Blush:_____

Bronzer:_____

Contour:_____

Highlight:_____

LIPS

Liner:_____

Gloss:_____

Color:_____

_____

CLIENT NAME

_____

MAKEUP ARTIST

_____

BRUSHES + TOOLS

_____

_____

_____

_____

_____

NOTES

_____

_____

_____

_____

_____

makeup face chart

LOOK NAME

_____

EYES

Brows:_____

Base:_____

Eye shadow:_____

_____

_____

Eyeliner:_____

Mascara:_____

Lashes:_____

FACE

Primer: _____

Concealer: _____

Foundation:_____

Powder:_____

Blush:_____

Bronzer: _____

Contour: _____

Highlight:_____

LIPS

Liner:_____

Gloss:_____

Color:_____

_____

CLIENT NAME

_____

MAKEUP ARTIST

_____

BRUSHES + TOOLS

NOTES

_____

_____

_____

_____

_____

_____

_____

_____

_____

_____

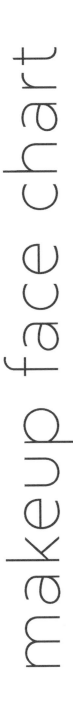

makeup face chart

LOOK NAME

_____

EYES

Brows:_____

Base:_____

Eye shadow:_____

_____

_____

Eyeliner:_____

Mascara:_____

Lashes:_____

FACE

Primer: _____

Concealer: _____

Foundation:_____

Powder:_____

Blush: _____

Bronzer: _____

Contour: _____

Highlight:_____

LIPS

Liner:_____

Gloss:_____

Color:_____

_____

CLIENT NAME

_____

MAKEUP ARTIST

_____

101

BRUSHES + TOOLS

_____

_____

_____

_____

_____

NOTES

_____

_____

_____

_____

_____

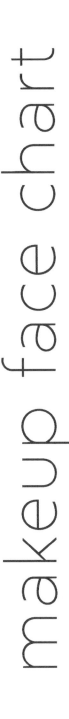

makeup face chart

LOOK NAME

_____

EYES

Brows:_____

Base:_____

Eye shadow:_____

_____

_____

Eyeliner:_____

Mascara:_____

Lashes:_____

FACE

Primer: _____

Concealer: _____

Foundation:_____

Powder:_____

Blush: _____

Bronzer: _____

Contour: _____

Highlight:_____

LIPS

Liner:_____

Gloss:_____

Color:_____

_____

CLIENT NAME

_____

MAKEUP ARTIST

_____

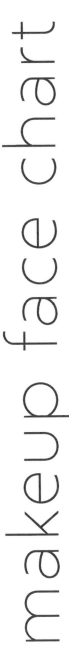

makeup face chart

LOOK NAME

_____

EYES

Brows:_____

Base:_____

Eye shadow:_____

_____

_____

Eyeliner:_____

Mascara:_____

Lashes:_____

FACE

Primer: _____

Concealer: _____

Foundation:_____

Powder:_____

Blush:_____

Bronzer: _____

Contour: _____

Highlight:_____

LIPS

Liner:_____

Gloss:_____

Color:_____

_____

CLIENT NAME

_____

MAKEUP ARTIST

_____

BRUSHES + TOOLS

_____

_____

_____

_____

_____

NOTES

_____

_____

_____

_____

_____

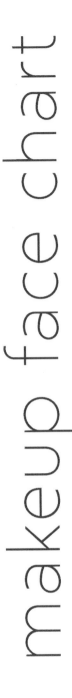

makeup face chart

LOOK NAME

_____

EYES

Brows:_____

Base:_____

Eye shadow:_____

_____

_____

Eyeliner:_____

Mascara:_____

Lashes:_____

FACE

Primer:_____

Concealer:_____

Foundation:_____

Powder:_____

Blush:_____

Bronzer:_____

Contour:_____

Highlight:_____

LIPS

Liner:_____

Gloss:_____

Color:_____

_____

CLIENT NAME

_____

MAKEUP ARTIST

_____

BRUSHES + TOOLS

_____

_____

_____

_____

_____

NOTES

_____

_____

_____

_____

_____

makeup face chart

LOOK NAME

_____

EYES

Brows:_____

Base:_____

Eye shadow:_____

_____

_____

Eyeliner:_____

Mascara:_____

Lashes:_____

FACE

Primer: _____

Concealer: _____

Foundation: _____

Powder:_____

Blush: _____

Bronzer: _____

Contour: _____

Highlight:_____

LIPS

Liner:_____

Gloss:_____

Color:_____

_____

CLIENT NAME

_____

MAKEUP ARTIST

_____

BRUSHES + TOOLS

_____

_____

_____

_____

_____

NOTES

_____

_____

_____

_____

_____

makeup face chart

LOOK NAME

_____

EYES

Brows:_____

Base:_____

Eye shadow:_____

_____

_____

Eyeliner:_____

Mascara:_____

Lashes:_____

FACE

Primer: _____

Concealer: _____

Foundation:_____

Powder:_____

Blush:_____

Bronzer:_____

Contour:_____

Highlight:_____

LIPS

Liner:_____

Gloss:_____

Color:_____

_____

CLIENT NAME

_____

MAKEUP ARTIST

_____

BRUSHES + TOOLS

_____

_____

_____

_____

_____

NOTES

_____

_____

_____

_____

_____

makeup face chart

LOOK NAME

_____

EYES

Brows:_____

Base:_____

Eye shadow:_____

_____

_____

Eyeliner:_____

Mascara:_____

Lashes:_____

FACE

Primer: _____

Concealer: _____

Foundation: _____

Powder:_____

Blush: _____

Bronzer: _____

Contour: _____

Highlight:_____

LIPS

Liner:_____

Gloss:_____

Color:_____

_____

CLIENT NAME

_____

MAKEUP ARTIST

_____

BRUSHES + TOOLS

_____

_____

_____

_____

_____

NOTES

_____

_____

_____

_____

_____

makeup face chart

LOOK NAME

_____

EYES

Brows:_____

Base:_____

Eye shadow:_____

_____

_____

Eyeliner:_____

Mascara:_____

Lashes:_____

FACE

Primer: _____

Concealer: _____

Foundation: _____

Powder:_____

Blush: _____

Bronzer: _____

Contour: _____

Highlight:_____

LIPS

Liner:_____

Gloss:_____

Color:_____

_____

CLIENT NAME

_____

MAKEUP ARTIST

_____

BRUSHES + TOOLS

_____

_____

_____

_____

_____

NOTES

_____

_____

_____

_____

_____

LOOK NAME

_____

EYES

Brows:_____

Base:_____

Eye shadow:_____

_____

_____

Eyeliner:_____

Mascara:_____

Lashes:_____

FACE

Primer: _____

Concealer: _____

Foundation:_____

Powder:_____

Blush: _____

Bronzer: _____

Contour: _____

Highlight:_____

LIPS

Liner:_____

Gloss:_____

Color:_____

_____

CLIENT NAME

_____

MAKEUP ARTIST

_____

BRUSHES + TOOLS

_____

_____

_____

_____

_____

NOTES

_____

_____

_____

_____

_____

makeup face chart

LOOK NAME

_____

EYES

Brows:_____

Base:_____

Eye shadow:_____

_____

_____

Eyeliner:_____

Mascara:_____

Lashes:_____

FACE

Primer: _____

Concealer: _____

Foundation:_____

Powder:_____

Blush: _____

Bronzer: _____

Contour: _____

Highlight:_____

LIPS

Liner:_____

Gloss:_____

Color:_____

_____

CLIENT NAME

_____

MAKEUP ARTIST

_____

BRUSHES + TOOLS

_____

_____

_____

_____

_____

NOTES

_____

_____

_____

_____

_____

makeup face chart

LOOK NAME

_____

EYES

Brows:_____

Base:_____

Eye shadow:_____

_____

_____

Eyeliner:_____

Mascara:_____

Lashes:_____

FACE

Primer: _____

Concealer: _____

Foundation: _____

Powder:_____

Blush: _____

Bronzer: _____

Contour: _____

Highlight:_____

LIPS

Liner:_____

Gloss:_____

Color:_____

_____

CLIENT NAME

_____

MAKEUP ARTIST

_____

BRUSHES + TOOLS

_____

_____

_____

_____

_____

NOTES

_____

_____

_____

_____

_____

makeup face chart

LOOK NAME

_____

EYES	FACE	LIPS
Brows:_____	Primer: _____	Liner:_____
Base:_____	Concealer: _____	Gloss:_____
Eye shadow:_____	Foundation:_____	Color:_____
_____	Powder:_____	_____
_____	Blush: _____	**CLIENT NAME**
Eyeliner:_____	Bronzer: _____	_____
Mascara:_____	Contour: _____	**MAKEUP ARTIST**
Lashes:_____	Highlight:_____	_____

BRUSHES + TOOLS

_____

_____

_____

_____

_____

NOTES

_____

_____

_____

_____

_____

makeup face chart

LOOK NAME

_____

EYES

Brows:_____

Base:_____

Eye shadow:_____

_____

_____

Eyeliner:_____

Mascara:_____

Lashes:_____

FACE

Primer: _____

Concealer: _____

Foundation:_____

Powder:_____

Blush:_____

Bronzer: _____

Contour: _____

Highlight:_____

LIPS

Liner:_____

Gloss:_____

Color:_____

_____

CLIENT NAME

_____

MAKEUP ARTIST

_____

makeup face chart

LOOK NAME

_____

EYES

Brows:_____

Base:_____

Eye shadow:_____

_____

_____

Eyeliner:_____

Mascara:_____

Lashes:_____

FACE

Primer: _____

Concealer: _____

Foundation:_____

Powder:_____

Blush:_____

Bronzer: _____

Contour: _____

Highlight:_____

LIPS

Liner:_____

Gloss:_____

Color:_____

_____

CLIENT NAME

_____

MAKEUP ARTIST

_____

BRUSHES + TOOLS

_____

_____

_____

_____

_____

NOTES

_____

_____

_____

_____

_____

makeup face chart

LOOK NAME

_____

EYES

Brows: _____

Base: _____

Eye shadow: _____

_____

_____

Eyeliner: _____

Mascara: _____

Lashes: _____

FACE

Primer: _____

Concealer: _____

Foundation: _____

Powder: _____

Blush: _____

Bronzer: _____

Contour: _____

Highlight: _____

LIPS

Liner: _____

Gloss: _____

Color: _____

_____

CLIENT NAME

_____

MAKEUP ARTIST

_____

makeup face chart

LOOK NAME

_____

EYES

Brows: _____

Base: _____

Eye shadow: _____

_____

_____

Eyeliner: _____

Mascara: _____

Lashes: _____

FACE

Primer: _____

Concealer: _____

Foundation: _____

Powder: _____

Blush: _____

Bronzer: _____

Contour: _____

Highlight: _____

LIPS

Liner: _____

Gloss: _____

Color: _____

_____

CLIENT NAME

_____

MAKEUP ARTIST

_____

BRUSHES + TOOLS

_____

_____

_____

_____

_____

NOTES

_____

_____

_____

_____

_____

makeup eye charts

LOOK NAME _____

EYE SHAPE _Almond_____

BROWS _____

LINER _____

EYE SHADOW _____

_____

LASHES _____

LOOK NAME _____

EYE SHAPE _Hooded_____

BROWS _____

LINER _____

EYE SHADOW _____

_____

LASHES _____

LOOK NAME _____

EYE SHAPE _Round_____

BROWS _____

LINER _____

EYE SHADOW _____

_____

LASHES _____

LOOK NAME _____

EYE SHAPE _Upturned_____

BROWS _____

LINER _____

EYE SHADOW _____

_____

LASHES _____

BRUSHES + TOOLS

NOTES

_____

_____

_____

_____

_____

_____

_____

_____

BRUSHES + TOOLS

NOTES

_____

_____

_____

_____

_____

_____

_____

_____

BRUSHES + TOOLS

NOTES

_____

_____

_____

_____

_____

_____

_____

_____

BRUSHES + TOOLS

NOTES

_____

_____

_____

_____

_____

_____

_____

_____

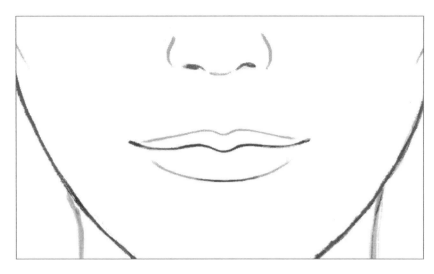

LOOK NAME _____

LIP SHAPE _Thin-upper_ _____

LINER _____

COLOR _____

GLOSS _____

NOTES _____

_____

_____

_____

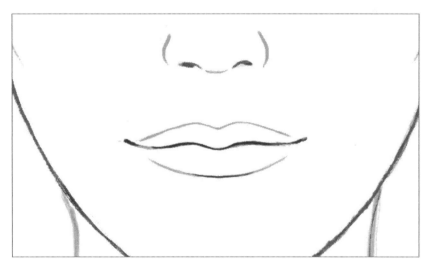

LOOK NAME _____

LIP SHAPE _Medium_ _____

LINER _____

COLOR _____

GLOSS _____

NOTES _____

_____

_____

_____

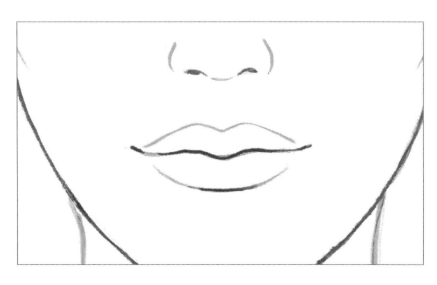

LOOK NAME _____

LIP SHAPE _Full_ _____

LINER _____

COLOR _____

GLOSS _____

NOTES _____

_____

_____

_____

BRUSHES + TOOLS

_____

_____

_____

_____

NOTES

_____

_____

_____

_____

BRUSHES + TOOLS

_____

_____

_____

_____

NOTES

_____

_____

_____

_____

BRUSHES + TOOLS

_____

_____

_____

_____

NOTES

_____

_____

_____

_____

makeup brow charts

NAME _____

BROW SHAPE _Straight_____

_____
_____
_____

NAME _____

BROW SHAPE _Round_____

_____
_____
_____

NAME _____

BROW SHAPE _Soft Angle_____

_____
_____
_____

NAME _____

BROW SHAPE _Sharp Angle_____

_____
_____
_____

NAME _____

BROW SHAPE _S-shape_____

_____
_____
_____

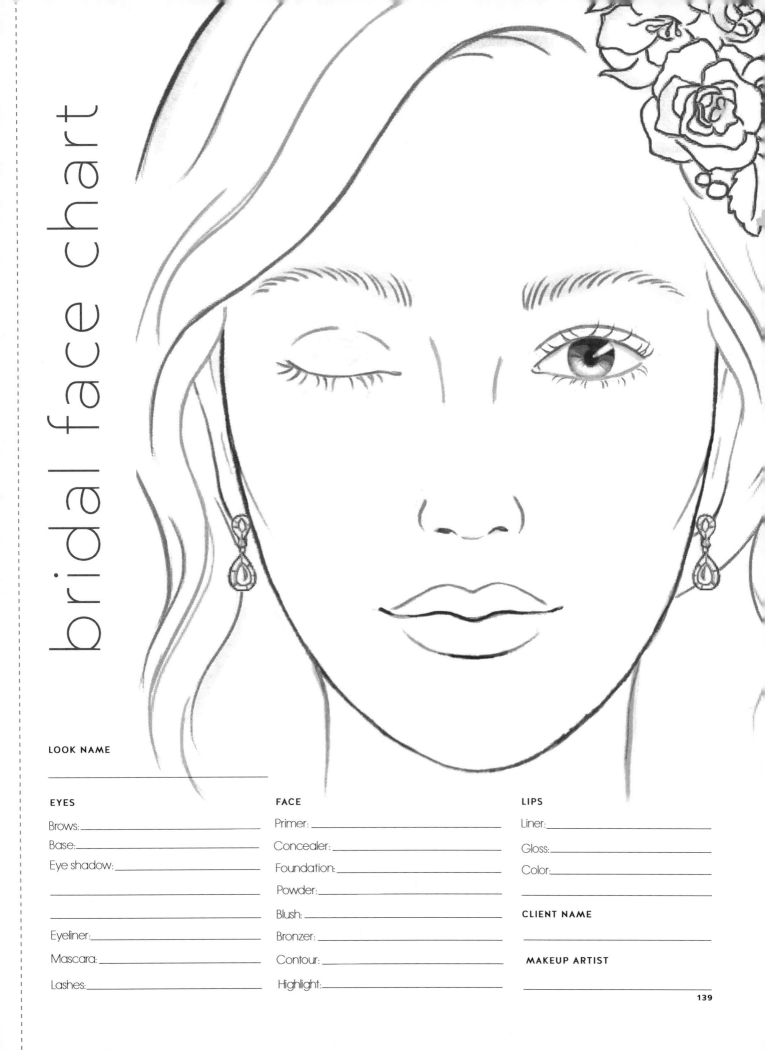

bridal face chart

LOOK NAME

_____

EYES

Brows:_____

Base:_____

Eye shadow:_____

_____

_____

Eyeliner:_____

Mascara:_____

Lashes:_____

FACE

Primer: _____

Concealer: _____

Foundation:_____

Powder:_____

Blush: _____

Bronzer: _____

Contour: _____

Highlight:_____

LIPS

Liner:_____

Gloss:_____

Color:_____

_____

CLIENT NAME

_____

MAKEUP ARTIST

_____

BRUSHES + TOOLS

_____

_____

_____

_____

_____

NOTES

_____

_____

_____

_____

_____

WEDDING DETAILS

_____

_____

_____

_____

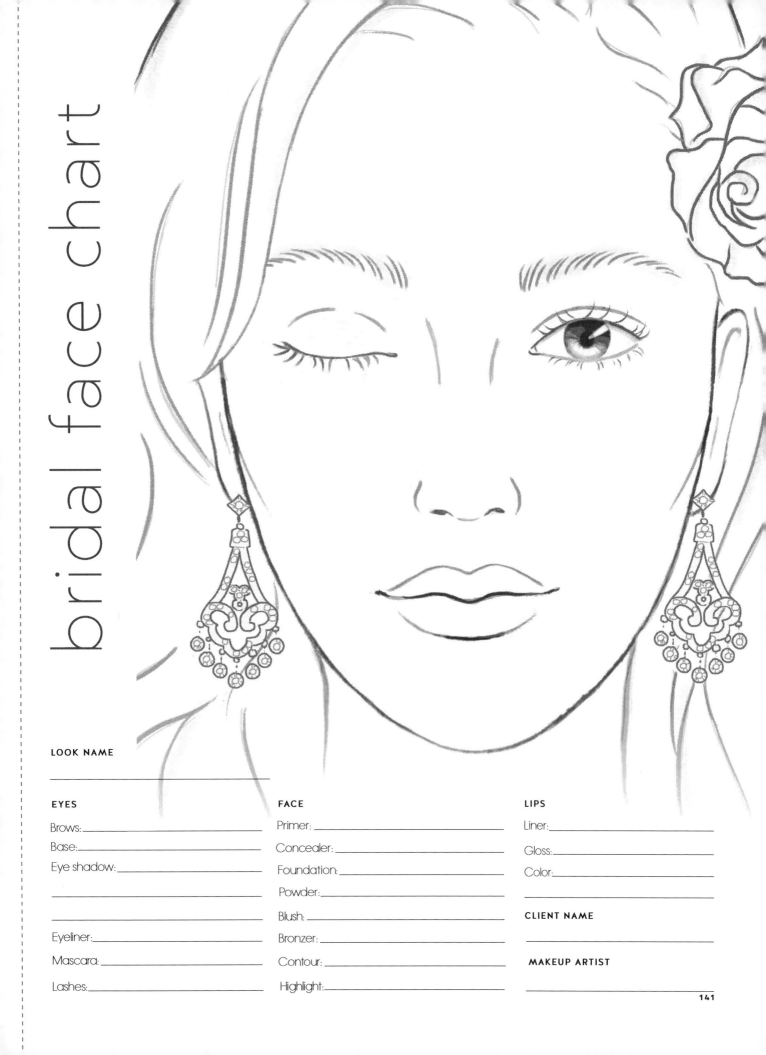

bridal face chart

LOOK NAME

_____

EYES

Brows:_____

Base:_____

Eye shadow:_____

_____

_____

Eyeliner:_____

Mascara:_____

Lashes:_____

FACE

Primer:_____

Concealer:_____

Foundation:_____

Powder:_____

Blush:_____

Bronzer:_____

Contour:_____

Highlight:_____

LIPS

Liner:_____

Gloss:_____

Color:_____

_____

CLIENT NAME

_____

MAKEUP ARTIST

_____

BRUSHES + TOOLS

_____

_____

_____

_____

_____

NOTES

_____

_____

_____

_____

_____

WEDDING DETAILS

_____

_____

_____

_____

Heart Face Shape
HIGHLIGHT + CONTOUR GUIDE

The highlight and contour method for a **Heart** face shape focuses on minimizing the width of the face and rounding out the strong angular structure of the jaw & point of chin.

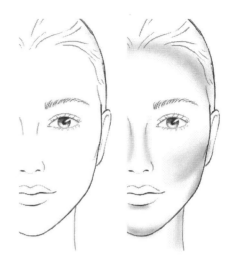

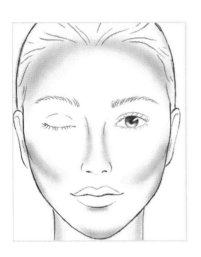

STEP 1: CONTOUR

Use dome blender brush and contour powder to shade:

Hairline
Under cheekbones (curved line)
Sides of neck (optional)

Define shading along **hairline & under cheekbones** with flat shader brush & contour powder.

Add shading to **sides of nose & under bottom lip** with pencil brush & contour powder. Also add contour along **tip of chin** to soften sharp angles.

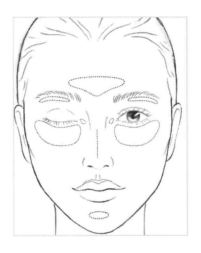

STEP 2: HIGHLIGHT + MID-TONE

Highlights are placed on the high points of the face. Use dome blender brush to apply highlight powder to (or leave areas blank if using white of paper as highlight)::

Forehead
Browbone
Inner eye corners
Under eyes
Cheekbones
Bridge of nose
Cupids bow
Center of chin

Apply mid-tone skincolor to blank areas between contour & highlight. Use small circular motions to create a seamless blend.

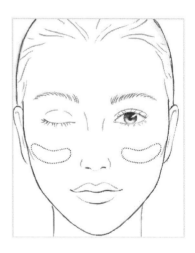

STEP 3: BLUSH

Balance sharp angle of jaw and point of chin with a curvy shape - similar to that of a kidney bean.

Apply blush with blender brush for added shape and natural flush of color.

sculpt + shape chart

LOOK NAME _____

FACE SHAPE: _Heart_ _____

HIGHLIGHT _____

CONTOUR _____

MID-TONE _____

FACE _____

_____

_____

_____

EYES _____

_____

_____

_____

LIPS _____

_____

_____

BRUSHES + TOOLS

_____

_____

_____

_____

_____

NOTES

_____

_____

_____

_____

_____

About the Creator

Gina M. Reyna, founder and owner of Colorista Books, has been a professional makeup artist since 2009. She is an Empire Beauty School graduate & has attended fine art classes at the Art Institute and the Academy of Art University San Francisco. Her experience as a makeup artist ranges from weddings & special events to editorial-style photography.

When Gina isn't working as a makeup artist, she spends her time creating content for makeup artists and beauty enthusiasts. Her first book, 'How to be a Professional Makeup Artist - A Comprehensive Guide for Beginners', was published in January of 2013. She has since then written 'The Complete Guide to Smokey Eyes' & created The Beauty Studio Collection of makeup charts.

If you have a question or comment for Gina, please send it to: gina@coloristabooks.com

To learn more visit us at:
COLORISTABOOKS.COM

Made in the USA
Las Vegas, NV
01 February 2024

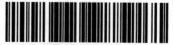

85167290R00083